CU00704240

Best
Keto Diet Cookbook
2021

Follow Mouthwatering Best Keto Recipes to Cook,

Increase Energy and Wow your Friends!

Mary Cue

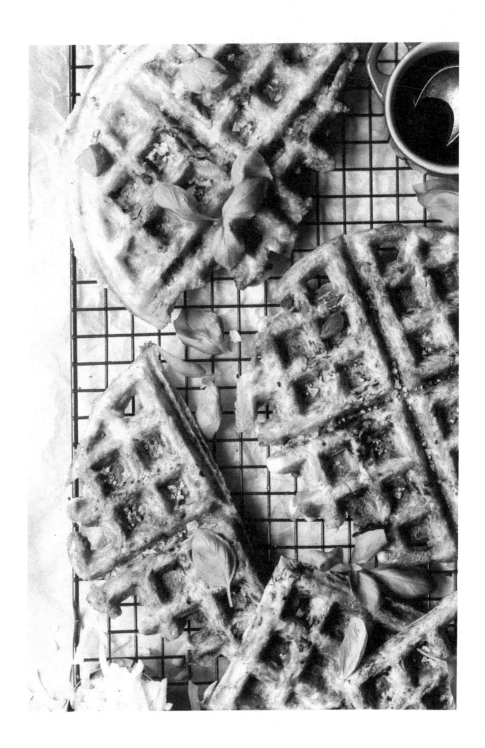

Table of Contents

© Copyright 2021 by Mary Cue

- All rights reserved.

The following Book is reproduced below with the goal of providing information that is as accurate and reliable as possible. Regardless, purchasing this Book can be seen as consent to the fact that both the publisher and the author of this book are in no way experts on the topics discussed within and that any recommendations or suggestions that are made herein are for entertainment purposes only. Professionals should be consulted as needed prior to undertaking any of the action endorsed herein.

This declaration is deemed fair and valid by both the American Bar Association and the Committee of Publishers Association and is legally binding throughout the United States.

Furthermore, the transmission, duplication, or reproduction of any of the following work including specific information will be considered an illegal act irrespective of if it is done electronically or in print. This extends to creating a secondary or tertiary copy of the work or a recorded copy and is only allowed with the express written consent from the Publisher. All additional right reserved.

The information in the following pages is broadly considered a truthful and accurate account of facts and as such, any inattention, use, or misuse of the information in question by the reader will render any resulting actions solely under their purview. There are no scenarios in which the publisher or the original author of this work can be in any fashion deemed liable for any hardship or damages that may befall them after undertaking information described herein.

Additionally, the information in the following pages is intended only for informational purposes and should thus be thought of as universal. As befitting its nature, it is presented without assurance regarding its prolonged validity or interim quality. Trademarks that are mentioned are done without written consent and can in no way be considered an endorsement from the trademark holder.

INTRODUCTION

So the Ketogenic Diet is all about reducing the amount of carbohydrates you eat. Does this mean you won't get the kind of energy you need for the day? Of course not! It only means that now, your body has to find other possible sources of energy. Do you know where they will be getting that energy?

Even before we talk about how to do keto – it's important to first consider why this particular diet works. What actually happens to your body to make you lose weight?

As you probably know, the body uses food as an energy source. Everything you eat is turned into energy, so that you can get up and do whatever you need to accomplish for the day. The main energy source is sugar so what happens is that you eat something, the body breaks it down into sugar, and the sugar is processed into energy. Typically, the "sugar" is taken directly from the food you eat so if you eat just the right amount of food, then your body is fueled for the whole day. If you eat too much, then the sugar is stored in your body – hence the accumulation of fat.

But what happens if you eat less food? This is where the Ketogenic Diet comes in. You see, the process of creating sugar from food is usually faster if the food happens to be rich in carbohydrates. Bread, rice, grain, pasta – all of these are carbohydrates and they're the easiest food types to turn into energy.

So here's the situation – you are eating less carbohydrates every day. To keep you energetic, the body breaks down the stored fat and turns them into molecules called ketone bodies. The process of turning the fat into ketone bodies is called "Ketosis" and obviously – this is where the name of the Ketogenic Diet comes from. The ketone bodies take the place of glucose in keeping you energetic. As long as you keep your carbohydrates reduced, the body will keep getting its energy from your body fat.

The Ketogenic Diet is often praised for its simplicity and when you look at it properly, the process is really straightforward. The Science behind the effectivity of the diet is also well-documented, and has been proven multiple times by different medical fields. For example, an article on Diet Review by Harvard provided a lengthy discussion on how the Ketogenic Diet works and why it is so effective for those who choose to use this diet.

But Fat Is the Enemy...Or Is It?

No – fat is NOT the enemy. Unfortunately, years of bad science told us that fat is something you have to avoid – but it's actually a very helpful thing for weight loss! Even before we move forward with this book, we'll have to discuss exactly what "healthy fats" are, and why they're actually the good guys. To do this, we need to make a distinction between the different kinds of fat. You've probably heard of them before and it is a little bit confusing at first. We'll try to go through them as simply as possible:

Saturated fat. This is the kind you want to avoid. They're also called "solid fat" because each molecule is packed with hydrogen atoms. Simply put, it's the kind of fat that can easily cause a blockage in your body. It can raise cholesterol levels and lead to heart problems or a stroke. Saturated fat is something you can find in meat, dairy products, and other processed food items. Now, you're probably wondering: isn't the Ketogenic Diet packed with saturated fat? The answer is: not necessarily. You'll find later in the recipes given that the Ketogenic Diet promotes primarily unsaturated fat or healthy fat. While there are definitely many meat recipes in the list, most of these recipes contain healthy fat sources.

Unsaturated Fat. These are the ones dubbed as healthy fat. They're the kind of fat you find in avocado, nuts, and other ingredients you usually find in Keto-friendly recipes. They're known to lower blood cholesterol and actually come in two types: polyunsaturated and monounsaturated. Both are good for your body but the benefits slightly vary, depending on what you're consuming.

Buffalo Chicken Sausage Balls

Preparation Time: 5 minutes

Cooking Time: 25 minutes

Servings: 2

Ingredients:

- Sausage Balls:

- 2 14-ox sausages, casings removed

- 2 cups almond flour

- 1 ½ cups shredded cheddar cheese

- ½ cup crumbled bleu cheese

- 1 tsp salt

- ½ tsp pepper

- Bleu Cheese Ranch Dipping Sauce:

- 1/3 cup mayonnaise

- 1/3 cup almond milk, unsweetened

- 2 cloves garlic, minced

- 1 tsp dried dill

- ½ tsp dried parsley

- ½ tsp salt

- ½ tsp pepper

- ¼ cup crumbled bleu cheese (or more, if desired)

Directions:

1. Preheat your oven at 35o degrees F.

2. Layer two baking sheets with wax paper and set them aside.

3. Mix sausage with cheddar cheese, almond flour, salt, pepper, and bleu cheese in a large bowl.

4. Make 1-inch balls out of this mixture and place them on the baking sheets.

5. Bake them for 25 minutes until golden brown.

6. Meanwhile, prepare the dipping sauce by whisking all of its ingredients in a bowl.

7. Serve the balls with this dipping sauce.

Nutrition: Calories: 183 Fat: 15 g Cholesterol 11 mg Sodium 31 mg Total carbohydrates 6.2 g Protein 4.5 g

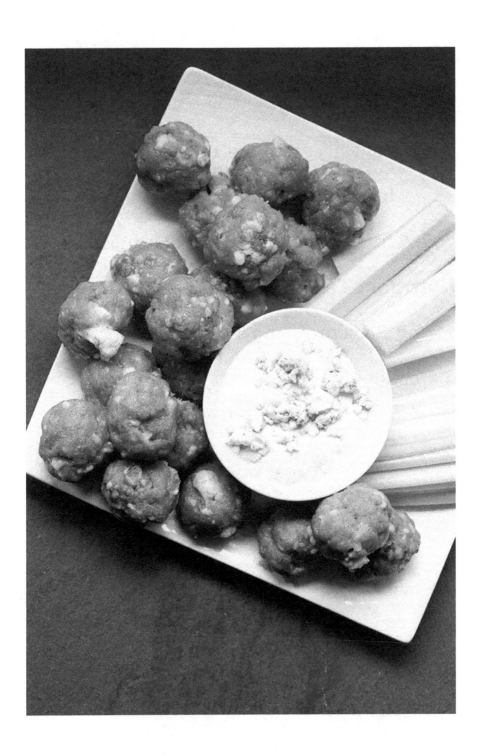

Brussels Sprouts Chips

Preparation Time: 5 minutes

Cooking Time: 15 minutes

Servings: 6

Ingredients:

- 1-pound Brussels sprouts, washed and dried
- 2 tbsp. extra virgin olive oil
- 1 tsp kosher salt

Directions:

1. Preheat your oven at 400 degrees F.
2. After peeling the sprouts off the stem, discard the outer leaves of the Brussel sprouts.
3. Separate all the leaves from one another and place them on a baking sheet.

4. Toss them with oil and salt thoroughly to coat them well.

5. Spread the leaves out on two greased baking sheets then bake them for 15 minutes until crispy.

6. Serve.

Nutrition: Calories: 188 Fat: 3 g Cholesterol: 101 Sodium: 54 mg Fiber 0.6 g Protein 5 g

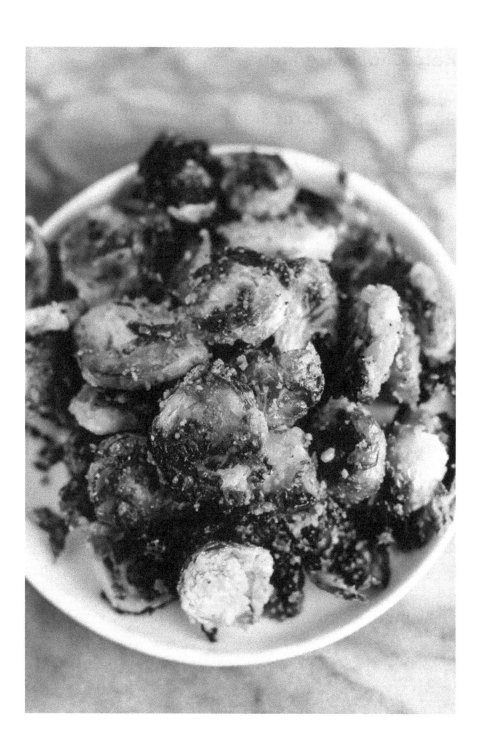

Keto Chocolate Mousse

Preparation Time: 5 minutes

Cooking Time: 0 minutes

Servings: 2

Ingredients:

- 1 cup heavy whipping cream
- ¼ cup unsweetened cocoa powder, sifted
- ¼ cup Swerve powdered sweetener
- 1 tsp vanilla extract
- ¼ tsp kosher salt

Directions:

1. Add cream to the bowl of an electric stand mixture and beat it until it forms peaks.
2. Stir in cocoa powder, vanilla, sweetener, and salt.
3. Mix well until smooth.

4. Refrigerate for 4 hours.

5. Serve.

Nutrition:

Calories: 153 Fat: 13 g

Cholesterol: 6.5 mg

Sodium: 81 mg

Sugar 1.4 g

Protein 5.8 g

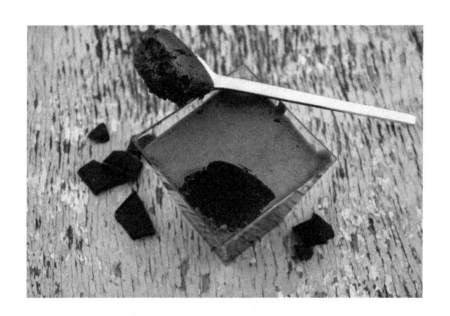

Keto Berry Mousse

Preparation Time: 5 minutes

Cooking Time: 0 minutes

Servings: 2

Ingredients:

- 2 cups heavy whipping cream

- 3 oz. fresh raspberries

- 2 oz. chopped pecans

- ½ lemon, zested

- ¼ tsp vanilla extract

Directions:

1. Beat cream in a bowl using a hand mixer until it forms peaks.

2. Stir in vanilla and lemon zest and mix well until incorporated.

3. Fold in nuts and berries and mix well.

4. Cover the mixture with plastic wrap and refrigerate for 3 hours.

5. Serve fresh.

Nutrition: Calories: 254 Fat: 9 g Cholesterol: 13 mg Sodium: 179 mg Sugar 1.2 g Protein 7.5 g

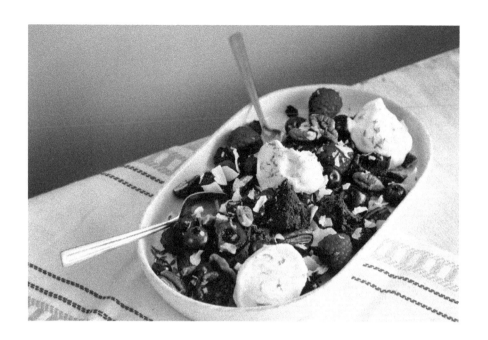

Peanut Butter Mousse

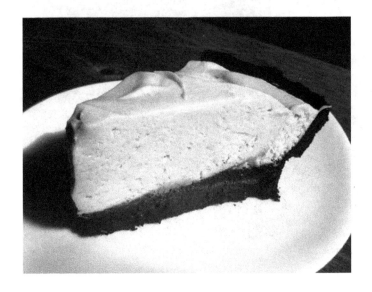

Preparation Time: 5 minutes

Cooking Time: 0 minutes

Servings: 4

Ingredients:

- ½ cup heavy whipping cream

- 4 oz. cream cheese, softened

- ¼ cup natural peanut butter

- ¼ cup powdered Swerve sweetener

- ½ tsp vanilla extract

Direction:

1. Beat ½ cup cream in a medium bowl with a hand mixer until it forms peaks.

2. Beat cream cheese with peanut butter in another bowl until creamy.

3. Stir in vanilla, a pinch of salt, and sweetener to the peanut butter mix and combine until smooth.

4. Fold in the prepared whipped cream and mix well until fully incorporated.

5. Divide the mousse into 4 serving glasses.

6. Garnish as desired.

7. Enjoy.

Nutrition: Calories: 290 Fat: 21.5 Cholesterol: 12 Sodium: 9 Protein: 6

Cookie Ice Cream

Preparation Time: 10 minutes

Cooking Time: 120 minutes

Servings: 2

Ingredients:

- Cookie Crumbs
- ¾ cup almond flour
- ¼ cup cocoa powder
- ¼ tsp baking soda
- ¼ cup erythritol
- ½ tsp vanilla extract
- 1 ½ tbsp. coconut oil, softened
- 1 large egg, room temperature
- Pinch of salt
- Ice Cream
- 2 ½ cups whipping cream

- 1 tbsp. vanilla extract

- ½ cup erythritol

- ½ cup almond milk, unsweetened

Directions:

1. Preheat your oven at 300 degrees F and layer a 9-inch baking pan with wax paper.

2. Whisk almond flour with baking soda, cocoa powder, salt, and erythritol in a medium bowl.

3. Stir in coconut oil and vanilla extract then mix well until crumbly.

4. Whisk in egg and mix well to form the dough.

5. Spread this dough in the prepared pan and bake for 20 minutes in the preheated oven.

6. Allow the crust to cool then crush it finely into crumbles.

7. Beat cream in a large bowl with a hand mixer until it forms a stiff peak.

8. Stir in erythritol and vanilla extract then mix well until fully incorporated.

9. Pour in milk and blend well until smooth.

10.   Add this mixture to an ice cream machine and churn as per the machine's instructions.

11.   Add cookie crumbles to the ice cream in the machine and churn again.

12.   Place the ice cream in a sealable container and freeze for 2 hours.

13.   Scoop out the ice cream and serve.

14.   Enjoy.

15.   *Note:* this recipe calls for an ice cream machine

Nutrition: Calories: 214 Fat: 19 Cholesterol: 15 Sodium: 12 Fiber: 2 Protein: 7

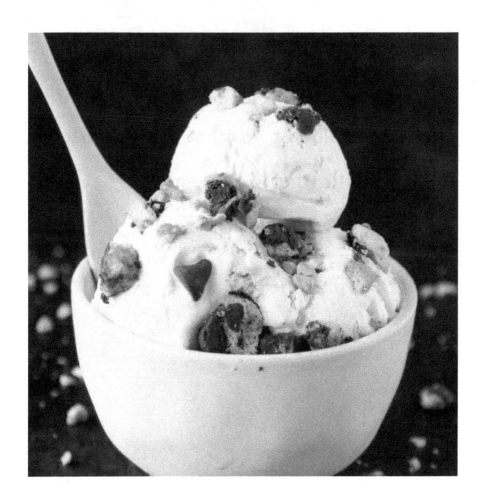

Mocha Ice Cream

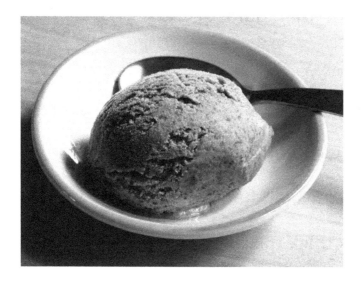

Preparation Time: 10 minutes

Cooking Time: 0 minutes

Servings: 2

Ingredients:

- 1 cup coconut milk

- ¼ cup heavy whipping cream

- 2 tbsp. erythritol

- 15 drops liquid stevia

- 2 tbsp. unsweetened cocoa powder

- 1 tbsp. instant coffee

- ¼ tsp xanthan gum

Directions:

1. Whisk everything except xanthan gum in a bowl using a hand mixer.

2. Slowly add xanthan gum and stir well to make a thick mixture.

3. Churn the mixture in an ice cream machine as per the machine's instructions.

4. Freeze it for 2 hours then garnish with mint and instant coffee.

5. Serve.

6. *Note:* this recipe calls for an ice cream machine

Nutrition: Calories: 267 Fat: 44.5 g Cholesterol: 153 mg Sodium: 217 mg

Raspberry Cream Fat Bombs

Preparation Time: 10 minutes

Cooking Time: 0 minutes

Servings: 2

Ingredients:

- 1 packet raspberry Jello (sugar-free)

- 1 tsp gelatin powder

- ½ cup of boiling water

- ½ cup heavy cream

Directions:

1. Mix Jello and gelatin in boiling water in a medium bowl.

2. Stir in cream slowly and mix it for 1 minute.

3. Divide this mixture into candy molds.

4. Refrigerate them for 30 minutes.

5. Enjoy.

Nutrition: Calories: 197 Fat: 19.2 g
Cholesterol: 11 mg Sodium: 78 mg

Cauliflower Tartar Bread

Preparation Time: 10 minutes

Cooking Time: 50 minutes

Servings: 4

Ingredients:

- 3 cup cauliflower rice
- 10 large eggs, yolks and egg whites separated
- ¼ tsp cream of tartar
- 1 ¼ cup coconut flour
- 1 ½ tbsp. gluten-free baking powder
- 1 tsp sea salt
- 6 tbsp. butter
- 6 cloves garlic, minced
- 1 tbsp. fresh rosemary, chopped
- 1 tbsp. fresh parsley, chopped

Directions:

1. Preheat your oven to 350 degrees F. Layer a 9x5-inch pan with wax paper.

2. Place the cauliflower rice in a suitable bowl and then cover it with plastic wrap.

3. Heat it for 4 minutes in the microwave. Heat more if the cauliflower isn't soft enough.

4. Place the cauliflower rice in a kitchen towel and squeeze it to drain excess water.

5. Transfer drained cauliflower rice to a food processor.

6. Add coconut flour, sea salt, baking powder, butter, egg yolks, and garlic. Blend until crumbly.

7. Beat egg whites with cream of tartar in a bowl until foamy.

8. Add egg white mixture to the cauliflower mixture and stir well with a spatula.

9. Fold in rosemary and parsley.

10.   Spread this batter in the prepared baking pan evenly.

11.   Bake it for 50 minutes until golden then allow it to cool.

Nutrition: Calories: 104 Fat: 8.9 g Cholesterol: 57 mg Sodium: 340 mg Carbohydrates: 4.7 g

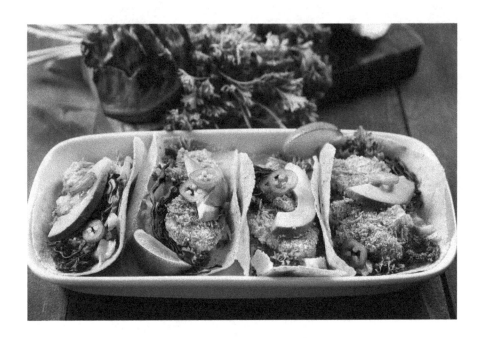

Buttery Skillet Flatbread

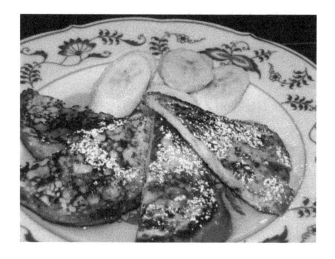

Preparation Time: 10 minutes

Cooking Time: 10 minutes

Servings: 4

Ingredients:

- 1 cup almond flour

- 2 tbsp. coconut flour

- 2 tsp xanthan gum

- ½ tsp baking powder

- ½ tsp salt

- 1 whole egg + 1 egg white

- 1 tbsp. water (if needed)

- 1 tbsp. oil, for frying

- 1 tbsp. melted butter, for brushing

Directions:

1. Mix xanthan gum with flours, salt, and baking powder in a suitable bowl.

2. Beat egg and egg white in a separate bowl then stir in the flour mixture.

3. Mix well until smooth. Add a tablespoon of water if the dough is too thick.

4. Place a large skillet over medium heat and heat oil.

Nutrition: Calories: 272 Fat: 18 Cholesterol: 6.1

Fluffy Bites

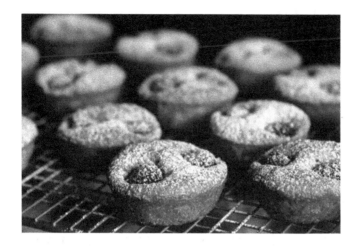

Preparation Time: 20 minutes

Cooking Time: 60 minutes

Servings: 12

Ingredients:

- 2 Teaspoons Cinnamon

- 2/3 Cup Sour Cream

- 2 Cups Heavy Cream

- 1 Teaspoon Scraped Vanilla Bean

- ¼ Teaspoon Cardamom

- 4 Egg Yolks

- Stevia to Taste

Directions:

1. Start by whisking your egg yolks until creamy and smooth.

2. Get out a double boiler, and add your eggs with the rest of your ingredients. Mix well.

3. Remove from heat, allowing it to cool until it reaches room temperature.

4. Refrigerate for an hour before whisking well.

5. Pour into molds, and freeze for at least an hour before serving.

Nutrition: Calories: 363 Protein: 2 Fat: 40 Carbohydrates: 1

Coconut Fudge

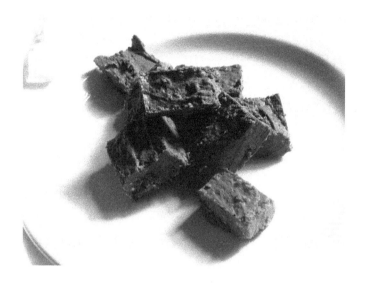

Preparation Time: 20 minutes

Cooking Time: 60 minutes

Servings: 12

Ingredients:

- 2 Cups Coconut Oil

- ½ Cup Dark Cocoa Powder

- ½ Cup Coconut Cream

- ¼ Cup Almonds, Chopped

- ¼ Cup Coconut, Shredded

- 1 Teaspoon Almond Extract

- Pinch of Salt

- Stevia to Taste

Directions:

1. Pour your coconut oil and coconut cream in a bowl, whisking with an electric beater until smooth. Once the mixture becomes smooth and glossy, do not continue.

2. Begin to add in your cocoa powder while mixing slowly, making sure that there aren't any lumps.

3. Add in the rest of your ingredients, and mix well.

4. Line a bread pan with parchment paper, and freeze until it sets.

5. Slice into squares before serving.

Nutrition: Calories: 172   Fat: 20

Carbohydrates: 3

Nutmeg Nougat

Preparation Time: 30 minutes

Cooking Time: 60 minutes

Servings: 12

Ingredients:

- 1 Cup Heavy Cream

- 1 Cup Cashew Butter

- 1 Cup Coconut, Shredded

- ½ Teaspoon Nutmeg

- 1 Teaspoon Vanilla Extract, Pure

- Stevia to Taste

Directions:

1. Melt your cashew butter using a double boiler, and then stir in your vanilla extract, dairy cream, nutmeg and stevia. Make sure it's mixed well.

2. Remove from heat, allowing it to cooldown before refrigerating it for a half hour.

3. Shape into balls, and coat with shredded coconut. Chill for at least two hours before serving.

Nutrition:

Calories: 341

Fat: 34

Carbohydrates: 5

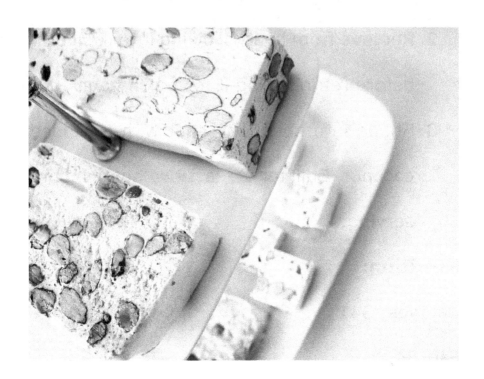

Sweet Almond Bites

Preparation Time: 30 minutes

Cooking Time: 90 minutes

Servings: 12

Ingredients:

- 18 Ounces Butter, Grass Fed

- 2 Ounces Heavy Cream

- ½ Cup Stevia

- 2/3 Cup Cocoa Powder

- 1 Teaspoon Vanilla Extract, Pure

- 4 Tablespoons Almond Butter

Direction:

1. Use a double boiler to melt your butter before adding in all of your remaining ingredients.

2. Place the mixture into molds, freezing for

two hours before serving.

Nutrition: Calories: 350 Protein: 2 Fat: 38

Strawberry Cheesecake Minis

Preparation Time: 30 minutes

Cooking Time: 120 minutes

Servings: 12

Ingredients:

- 1 Cup Coconut Oil

- 1 Cup Coconut Butter

- ½ Cup Strawberries, Sliced

- ½ Teaspoon Lime Juice

- 2 Tablespoons Cream Cheese, Full Fat

- Stevia to Taste

Directions:

1. Blend your strawberries together.

2. Soften your cream cheese, and then add in your coconut butter.

3. Combine all ingredients together, and then pour your mixture into silicone molds.

4. Freeze for at least two hours before serving.

Nutrition: Calories: 372 Protein: 1   Fat: 41 Carbohydrates: 2

Cocoa Brownies

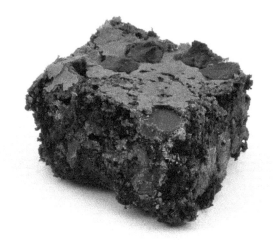

Preparation Time: 10 minutes

Cooking Time: 30 minutes

Servings: 12

Ingredients:

- 1 Egg

- 2 Tablespoons Butter, Grass Fed

- 2 Teaspoons Vanilla Extract, Pure

- ¼ Teaspoon Baking Powder

- ¼ Cup Cocoa Powder

- 1/3 Cup Heavy Cream

- ¾ Cup Almond Butter

- Pinch Sea Salt

Directions:

1. Break your egg into a bowl, whisking until smooth.

2. Add in all of your wet ingredients, mixing well.

3. Mix all dry ingredients into a bowl.

4. Sift your dry ingredients into your wet ingredients, mixing to form a batter.

5. Get out a baking pan, greasing it before pouring in your mixture.

6. Heat your oven to 350 and bake for twenty-five minutes.

7. Allow it to cool before slicing and serve room temperature or warm.

Nutrition: Calories: 184 Protein: 1 Fat: 20 Carbohydrates: 1

Chocolate Orange Bites

Preparation Time: 20 minutes

Cooking Time: 120 minutes

Servings: 6

Ingredients:

- 10 Ounces Coconut Oil
- 4 Tablespoons Cocoa Powder
- ¼ Teaspoon Blood Orange Extract
- Stevia to Taste

Directions:

1. Melt half of your coconut oil using a double boiler, and then add in your stevia and orange extract.

2. Get out candy molds, pouring the mixture into it. Fill each mold halfway, and then place in the fridge until they set.

3. Melt the other half of your coconut oil, stirring in your cocoa powder and stevia, making sure that the mixture is smooth with no lumps.

4. Pour into your molds, filling them up all the way, and then allow it to set in the fridge before serving.

Nutrition: Calories: 188 Protein: 1 Fat: 21 Carbohydrates: 5

Caramel Cones

Preparation Time: 25 minutes

Cooking Time: 120 minutes

Servings: 6

Ingredients:

- 2 Tablespoons Heavy Whipping Cream

- 2 Tablespoons Sour Cream

- 1 Tablespoon Caramel Sugar

- 1 Teaspoon Sea Salt, Fine

- 1/3 Cup Butter, Grass Fed

- 1/3 Cup Coconut Oil

- Stevia to Taste

Directions:

1. Soften your coconut oil and butter, mixing together.

2. Mix all ingredients together to form a batter, and ten place them in molds.

3. Top with a little salt, and keep refrigerated until serving.

Nutrition: Calories: 100 Fat: 12 Grams Carbohydrates: 1

Cinnamon Bites

Preparation Time: 20 minutes

Cooking Time: 95 minutes

Servings: 6

Ingredients:

- 1/8 Teaspoon Nutmeg

- 1 Teaspoon Vanilla Extract

- ¼ Teaspoon Cinnamon

- 4 Tablespoons Coconut Oil

- ½ Cup Butter, Grass Fed

- 8 Ounces Cream Cheese

- Stevia to Taste

Directions:

1. Soften your coconut oil and butter, mixing in your cream cheese.

2. Add all of your remaining ingredients, and

mix well.

3. Pour into molds, and freeze until set.

Nutrition: Calories: 178 Protein: 1 Fat: 19

Sweet Chai Bites

Preparation Time: 20 minutes

Cooking Time: 45 minutes

Servings: 6

Ingredients:

- 1 Cup Cream Cheese

- 1 Cup Coconut Oil

- 2 Ounces Butter, Grass Fed

- 2 Teaspoons Ginger

- 2 Teaspoons Cardamom

- 1 Teaspoon Nutmeg

- 1 Teaspoon Cloves

- 1 Teaspoon Vanilla Extract, Pure

- 1 Teaspoon Darjeeling Black Tea

- Stevia to Taste

Directions:

1. Melt your coconut oil and butter before adding in your black tea. Allow it to set for one to two minutes.

2. Add in your cream cheese, removing your mixture from heat.

3. Add in all of your spices, and stir to combine.

4. Pour into molds, and freeze before serving.

Nutrition: Calories: 178 Protein: 1 *Fat:* 19

Easy Vanilla Bombs

Preparation Time: 20 minutes

Cooking Time: 45 minutes

Servings: 14

Ingredients:

- 1 Cup Macadamia Nuts, Unsalted
- ¼ Cup Coconut Oil / ¼ Cup Butter
- 2 Teaspoons Vanilla Extract, Sugar Free
- 20 Drops Liquid Stevia
- 2 Tablespoons Erythritol, Powdered

Directions:

1. Pulse your macadamia nuts in a blender, and then combine all of your ingredients together. Mix well.
2. Get out mini muffin tins with a tablespoon and a half of the mixture.

3. Refrigerate it for a half hour before serving.

Nutrition: Calories: 125 Fat: 5 Carbohydrates: 5

Marinated Eggs

Preparation Time: 2 hours and 10 minutes

Cooking Time: 7 minutes

Servings: 4

Ingredients:

- 6 eggs

- 1 and ¼ cups water

- ¼ cup unsweetened rice vinegar 2 tablespoons coconut aminos

- Salt and black pepper to the taste 2 garlic cloves, minced

- 1 teaspoon stevia 4 ounces cream cheese

- 1 tablespoon chives, chopped

Directions:

1. Put the eggs in a pot, add water to cover, bring to a boil over medium heat, cover and cook for 7 minutes.

2. Rinse eggs with cold water and leave them aside to cool down.

3. In a bowl, mix 1 cup water with coconut aminos, vinegar, stevia and garlic and whisk well.

4. Put the eggs in this mix, cover with a kitchen towel and leave them aside for 2 hours rotating from time to time.

5. Peel eggs, cut in halves and put egg yolks in a bowl.

6. Add ¼ cup water, cream cheese, salt, pepper and chives and stir well.

7. Stuff egg whites with this mix and serve them.

8. Enjoy!

Nutrition: Calories: 289 kcal Protein: 15.86 g Fat: 22.62 g Carbohydrates: 4.52 g Sodium: 288 mg

Sausage and Cheese Dip

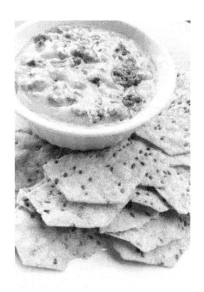

Preparation Time: 10 minutes

Cooking Time: 130 minutes

Servings: 28

Ingredients:

- 8 ounces cream cheese

- A pinch of salt and black pepper

- 16 ounces sour cream

- 8 ounces pepper jack cheese, chopped

- 15 ounces canned tomatoes mixed with habaneros

- 1 pound Italian sausage, ground

- ¼ cup green onions, chopped

Directions:

1. Heat up a pan over medium heat, add sausage, stir and cook until it browns.

2. Add tomatoes mix, stir and cook for 4 minutes more.

3. Add a pinch of salt, pepper and the green onions, stir and cook for 4 minutes.

4. Spread pepper jack cheese on the bottom of your slow cooker.

5. Add cream cheese, sausage mix and sour cream, cover and cook on High for 2 hours.

6. Uncover your slow cooker, stir dip, transfer to a bowl and serve.

7. Enjoy!

Nutrition: Calories: 132 kcal Protein: 6.79 g Fat: 9.58 g Carbohydrates: 6.22 g Sodium: 362 mg

Tasty Onion and Cauliflower Dip.

Preparation Time: 20 minutes

Cooking Time: 30 minutes

Servings: 24

Ingredients:

- 1 and ½ cups chicken stock

- 1 cauliflower head, florets separated

- ¼ cup mayonnaise

- ½ cup yellow onion, chopped

- ¾ cup cream cheese

- ½ teaspoon chili powder

- ½ teaspoon cumin, ground

- ½ teaspoon garlic powder

- Salt and black pepper to the taste

Directions:

1. Put the stock in a pot, add cauliflower and onion, heat up over medium heat and cook for 30 minutes.

2. Add chili powder, salt, pepper, cumin and garlic powder and stir.

3. Also add cream cheese and stir a bit until it melts.

4. Blend using an immersion blender and mix with the mayo.

5. Transfer to a bowl and keep in the fridge for 2 hours before you serve it.

6. Enjoy!

Nutrition: Calories: 40 kcal Protein: 1.23 g Fat: 3.31 g Carbohydrates: 1.66 g Sodium: 72 mg

Pesto Crackers

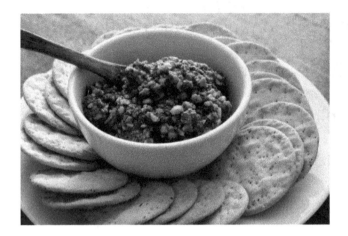

Preparation Time: 10 minutes

Cooking Time: 17 minutes

Servings: 6

Ingredients

- ½ teaspoon baking powder

- Salt and black pepper to the taste

- 1 and ¼ cups almond flour ¼ teaspoon basil, dried 1 garlic clove, minced

- 2 tablespoons basil pesto

- A pinch of cayenne pepper

- 3 tablespoons ghee

Directions:

1. In a bowl, mix salt, pepper, baking powder and almond flour.

2. Add garlic, cayenne and basil and stir.

3. Add pesto and whisk.

4. Also add ghee and mix your dough with your finger.

5. Spread this dough on a lined baking sheet, introduce in the oven at 325 degrees F and bake for 17 minutes.

6. Leave aside to cool down, cut your crackers and serve them as a snack.

7. Enjoy!

Nutrition: Calories: 9 kcal Protein: 0.41 g Fat:

0.14 g Carbohydrates: 1.86 g Sodium: 2 mg

Coconut Milk Latte

Preparation Time: 5 minutes

Cooking Time: 5 minutes

Servings: 2

Ingredients:

- 3 cups prepared hot coffee

- 1/2 cup coconut cream

- Dash of cinnamon

Directions:

1. Empty the espresso into a blender alongside the coconut milk.

2. Mix on medium-high for about a moment, or until the coconut milk is totally fused.

3. Fill a mug or serve over ice. You can spoon the foamed coconut milk on top for some "froth".

4. Change the measure of coconut milk to your taste buds... you may need pretty much.

Nutrition: Calories 114 Fat 12g Carbs 1g Sugar 2g Protein 1g

Chamomile Mint Tea Recipe

Preparation Time: 5minutes

Cooking Time: 0 minutes

Servings: 1

Ingredients:

- 1 tsp chamomile flowers

- 1 tsp peppermint leaves

- 1 cup (240 ml) boiling water

Directions:

1. Combine the chamomile and peppermint to a tea kettle

2. Mix for 4-5mins, discharges the herbs and drink.

Nutrition: Calories: 159 Fat 18g Carbs 9g Sugar 4g Protein 8g

Keto Iced Apple Green Tea

Preparation Time: 5 minutes

Cooking Time: 0 minutes

Servings: 2

Ingredients:

- 1 cup of brewed green tea

- 1 cup ice

- 1 tsp apple cider vinegar

- Stevie

Directions:

1. Mix the green tea with high temp water for 2-3 minutes.

2. Add every one of the **Ingredients:** to a blender and mix well.

Nutrition: Calories 190 Fat 17g Carbs 10g Sugar 1g Protein 3g

APPETIZERS

Bacon Peppers

Preparation Time: 15 minutes

Cooking Time: 6 minutes

Servings: 2

Ingredients:

- 2 jalapenos

- 1 oz. bacon, chopped, fried

- 1 teaspoon green onions, chopped

- 1 tablespoon coconut cream

- 2 oz. Cheddar cheese, shredded

Directions:

1. Trim the jalapenos and remove the seeds.

2. In the mixing bowl, mix up chopped bacon, green onions, coconut cream, and shredded cheese.

3. Fill the jalapenos with the bacon mixture.

4. Heat up the instant pot on saute mode for 5 minutes.

5. Put the jalapenos in the instant pot and cook them for 3 minutes from each side.

Nutrition: Calories 213 Fat 17.2 Fiber 0.6 Carbs 1.9 Protein 12.7

Fat Bombs

Preparation Time: 10 minutes

Cooking Time: 10 minutes

Servings: 3

Ingredients:

- 3 eggs

- 3 bacon slices

- ½ teaspoon cayenne pepper

- 2 tablespoons cream cheese

- ½ teaspoon salt

Directions:

1. Put the bacon in the instant pot and cook it on saute mode for 3 minutes from each side.

2. Then chop the bacon and put it in the bowl.

3. Crack the eggs in the instant pot and whisk gently.

4. Cook the eggs for 5 minutes on manual mode (high pressure). Make a quick pressure release.

5. Then transfer the cooked eggs in the bowl with bacon and shred.

6. Add cayenne pepper, cream cheese, and salt. Stir well.

7. Make the medium size bombs.

Nutrition: Calories 190 Fat 14.7 Fiber 0.1 Carbs 1 Protein 13.1

Chicken Celery Sticks

Preparation Time: 15 minutes

Cooking Time: 15 minutes

Servings: 4

Ingredients:

- 14 oz. chicken breast, skinless, boneless

- 1 cup of water

- 1 teaspoon salt

- ½ teaspoon onion powder

- 4 celery stalks

- 1 teaspoon Keto mayo

Directions:

1. Put the chicken breast in the instant pot.

2. Add water, salt, and onion powder.

3. Cook the chicken on manual mode (high pressure) for 15 minutes. Allow the natural pressure release for 6 minutes.

4. Remove the cooked chicken from the instant pot and shred it.

5. Add Keto mayo and stir well.

6. Fill the celery stalks with shredded chicken.

Nutrition: Calories 118 Fat 2.6 Fiber 0.3 Carbs 0.9 Protein 21.2

Reuben Pickles

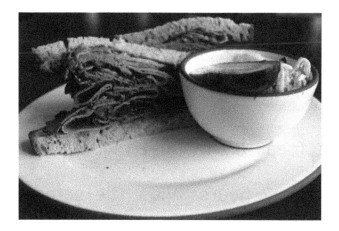

Preparation Time: 20 minutes

Cooking Time: 2 hours

Servings: 6

Ingredients:

- 1-pound corned beef brisket

- 2 cups of water

- 1 cup pickled cucumbers

- 2 oz. provolone cheese, sliced

Directions:

1. Put corned beef brisket and water in the instant pot.

2. Cook the meat on manual mode (high pressure) for 2 hours. Allow the natural pressure release for 10 minutes.

3. Then remove the meat from water and slice it.

4. Make the Reuben pickles: pin the meat piece, pickled cucumber, and provolone cheese together to get the small bites.

Nutrition: Calories 164 Fat 12 Fiber 0.1 Carbs 0.8 Protein 12.7

Parmesan Balls with Greens

Preparation Time: 10 minutes

Cooking Time: 20 minutes

Servings: 4

Ingredients:

- 3 oz. Parmesan, grated

- 1 cup ground chicken

- 1 tablespoon chives, chopped

- 1 teaspoon cayenne pepper

- ¼ cup chicken broth

- 1 teaspoon coconut oil, softened

Directions:

1. Heat up coconut oil in the instant pot on saute mode.

2. Add ground chicken, cayenne pepper, chives, and chicken broth.

3. Close the lid and cook the chicken on manual mode (high pressure) for 15 minutes.

4. Then make a quick pressure release and open the lid.

5. Add Parmesan and stir the chicken mixture well.

6. Make the balls from the cooked mixture and cool them for 10 minutes before serving.

Nutrition: Calories 149 Fat 8.5 Fiber 0.1 Carbs 1.1 Protein 17.3

Cheese Stuffed Shishito Peppers

Preparation Time: 20 minutes

Cooking Time: 7 minutes

Servings: 4

Ingredients:

- 8 oz. shishito peppers

- 1 cup Cheddar cheese, shredded

- 4 tablespoons cream cheese

- 1 tablespoon fresh parsley, chopped

- ¼ teaspoon minced garlic

- 1 tablespoon butter, melted

- 1 cup water, for cooking

Directions:

1. Cut the ends of the peppers and remove the seeds.

2. After this, in the mixing bowl mix up shredded cheese, cream cheese, parsley, and minced garlic.

3. Then fill the peppers with cheese mixture and put in the baking mold.

4. Sprinkle the peppers with melted butter.

5. After this, pour water and insert the steamer rack.

6. Place the mold with peppers on the rack. Close and seal the lid.

7. Cook the meal on manual (high pressure) for 7 minutes. Allow the natural pressure release for 5 minutes

Nutrition: Calories 194 Fat 15.7 Fiber 2.6 Carbs 4.5 Protein 9.1

Roasted Tomatillos

Preparation Time: 10 minutes

Cooking Time: 10 minutes

Servings: 4

Ingredients:

- tablespoon Italian seasonings

- 4 tomatillos, sliced

- 4 teaspoons olive oil

- 4 tablespoons water

Directions:

1. Sprinkle the tomatillos with Italian seasoning.

2. Then pour the olive oil in the instant pot and heat it up on saute mode for 1 minute.

3. Put the tomatillos in the instant pot in one layer and cook them for 2 minutes from each side.

4. Then add water and close the lid.

5. Saute the vegetables for 3 minutes more.

Nutrition: Calories 51 Fat 5 Fiber 0.7 Carbs 2 Protein 0.3

Chicken & Chinese Cabbage Salad

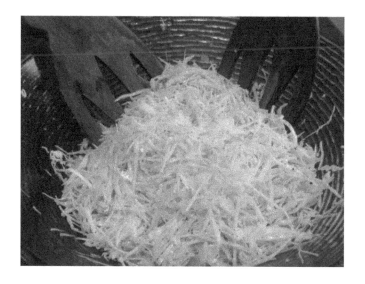

Preparation Time: 15 minutes

Cooking Time: 10 minutes

Servings: 4

Ingredients:

- 12 oz. chicken fillet, chopped

- 1 teaspoon Cajun seasonings

- 1 tablespoon coconut oil

- 1 cup Chinese cabbage, chopped

- 1 tablespoon avocado oil

- 1 teaspoon sesame seeds

Directions:

1. Sprinkle the chopped chicken with Cajun seasonings and put in the instant pot.

2. Add coconut oil and cook the chicken on saute mode for 10 minutes. Stir it from time to time with the help of a spatula.

3. When the chicken is cooked, transfer it in the salad bowl.

4. Add Chinese cabbage, avocado oil, and sesame seeds.

5. Mix up the salad.

Nutrition: Calories 202 Fat 10.6 Fiber 0.4 Carbs 0.8 Protein 25

Cauliflower Fritters

Preparation Time: 10 minutes

Cooking Time: 10 minutes

Servings: 4

Ingredients:

- 1 cup cauliflower, boiled

- 2 oz. Cheddar cheese, shredded

- 2 tablespoons almond flour

- ½ teaspoon garlic powder

- 2 eggs, beaten

- 1 tablespoon avocado oil

Directions:

1. Mash the cauliflower and mix it up with Cheddar cheese, almond flour, garlic powder, and eggs.

2. Heat up the avocado oil on saute mode for 1 minute.

3. Meanwhile, make the fritters from the cauliflower mixture.

4. Put them in the hot oil and cook for 3 minutes from each side.

Nutrition: Calories 122 Fat 9 Fiber 1.2 Carbs 2.9 Protein 7.7

Matcha Smoothie

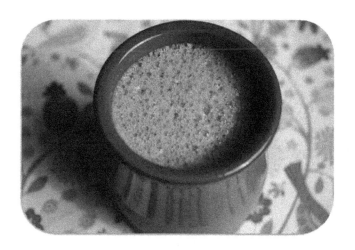

Preparation Time: 10 minutes

Cooking Time: 10 minutes

Servings: 2

Ingredients:

- 2 tablespoons chia seeds

- 2 teaspoons matcha green tea powder

- ½ teaspoon fresh lemon juice

- ½ teaspoon xanthan gum

- 10 drops liquid stevia

- 4 tablespoons plain Greek yogurt

- 1½ cups unsweetened almond milk

- ¼ cup ice cubes

Directions:

1. In a blender, put all the listed **Ingredients:** and pulse until creamy.

2. Pour the smoothie into two glasses and serve immediately.

Nutrition: Calories 85 Net Carbs 3.5 g Total Fat 5.5 g Saturated Fat 0.8 g Cholesterol 2 mg Sodium 174 mg

Total Carbs 7.6 g Fiber 4.1 g Sugar 2.2 g Protein 4 g

Creamy Spinach Smoothie

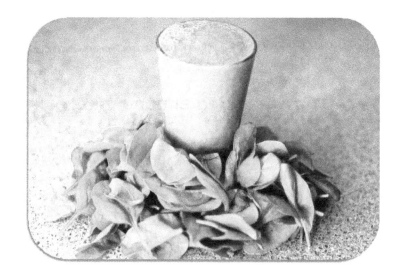

Preparation Time: 10 minutes

Cooking Time: 10 minutes

Servings: 2

Ingredients:

- 2 cups fresh baby spinach

- 1 tablespoon almond butter

- 1 tablespoon chia seeds

- 1/8 teaspoon ground cinnamon

- Pinch of ground cloves

- ½ cup heavy cream

- 1 cup unsweetened almond milk

- ½ cup ice cubes

Directions:

1. In a blender, put all the listed **Ingredients:** and pulse until creamy.

2. Pour the smoothie into two glasses and serve immediately.

Nutrition: Calories 195 Net Carbs 2.8 g Total Fat 18.8 g Saturated Fat 7.5 g Cholesterol 41 mg Sodium 126 mg Total Carbs 6.1 g Fiber 3.3 g Sugar 0.5 g Protein 4.5 g

CONCLUSION

The things to watch out for when coming off keto are weight gain, bloating, more energy, and feeling hungry. The weight gain is nothing to freak out over; perhaps, you might not even gain any. It all depends on your diet, how your body processes carbs, and, of course, water weight. The length of your keto diet is a significant factor in how much weight you have lost, which is caused by the reduction of carbs. The bloating will occur because of the reintroduction of fibrous foods and your body getting used to digesting them again. The bloating van lasts for a few days to a few weeks. You will feel like you have more energy because carbs break down into glucose, which is the body's primary source of fuel. You may also notice better brain function and the ability to work out more.

Whether you have met your weight loss goals, your life changes, or you simply want to eat whatever you want again. You cannot just suddenly start consuming carbs again for it will shock your system. Have an idea of what you want to allow back into your consumption slowly. Be familiar with portion sizes and stick to that amount of carbs for the first few times you eat post-keto. Start with non-processed carbs like whole grain, beans, and fruits. Start slow and see how your body responds before resolving to add carbs one meal at a time.

The ketogenic diet is the ultimate tool you can use to plan your future. Can you picture being more involved, more productive and efficient, and more relaxed and energetic? That future is possible for you, and it does not have to be a complicated process to achieve that vision. You can choose right now to be healthier and slimmer and more fulfilled tomorrow. It is possible with the ketogenic diet. It does not just improve your physical health but your mental and emotional health as well. This diet improves your health holistically. Do not give up now as there will be quite a few days where you may think to yourself, "Why am I doing this?" and to answer that, simply focus on the goals you wish to achieve. A good diet enriched with all the proper nutrients is our best shot of achieving an active metabolism and efficient lifestyle. A lot of people think that the Keto diet is simply for people who are interested in losing weight. You will find that it is quite the opposite. There are intense keto diets where only 5 percent of the diet comes from carbs, 20 percent is from protein, and 75 percent is from fat. But even a modified version of this which involves consciously choosing foods low in carbohydrate and high in healthy fats is good enough. Thanks for reading this book. I hope it has provided you with enough insight to get you going. Don't put off getting started. The sooner you begin this diet, the sooner you'll start to notice an improvement in your health and well-being.